UNDERSTANDING THE POWER OF HARMONY:

Nurturing parenting, Building lasting relationships, knowing how to manage your family, work and life.

Daniel Tucker

Introduction

INTRODUCTION

Embracing the Journey of Parenthood and Relationships

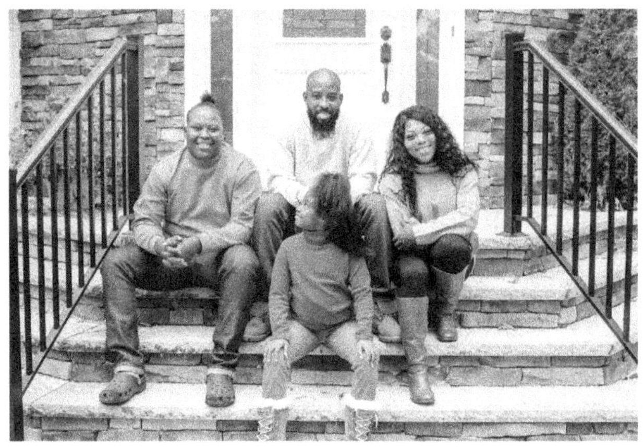

Welcome to the profound exploration of life's most rewarding and intricate odyssey: the journey of parenthood and relationships.

In the tapestry of existence, few threads weave a more intricate and meaningful pattern than the bonds we forge with our children and partners.

This book is an invitation to embark on a voyage where the compass is love, the map is understanding, and the destination is a harmonious haven called home. Whether you are a new parent navigating the uncharted waters of early parenthood or a seasoned traveler seeking to deepen the connections in your family and relationships, this guide is a companion for all stages of life.

We will delve into the foundations of family, navigate the ebbs and flows of parenthood, and explore the art of fostering enduring connections with our partners.

Together, we will uncover the secrets of effective communication, discover the delicate balance between personal growth and family life, and learn the art of resilience when faced with the inevitable storms of life.

As we journey through these pages, may you find inspiration, guidance, and practical insights to create a home where love roots run deep. Embrace the challenges, savor the joys, and relish in the growth that comes from nurturing a thriving family and fulfilling relationships.

So, let us embark on this adventure together, embracing the beauty and complexity of the journey of parenthood and relationships—a journey that promises growth, joy, and the creation of lasting memories.

CHAPTER 1

Foundations of family

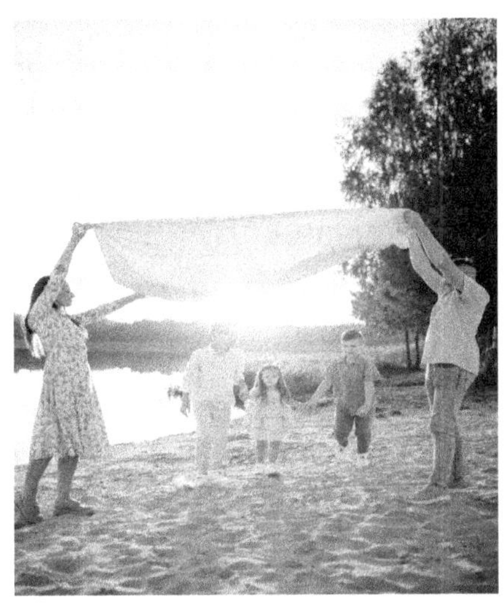

Having a strong nuclear family is significant, and to accomplish one, families should make major areas of strength for an establishment.

Here are ways families foster solid groundworks to expand upon and help them through when the times get hard?

• Be Available

Remaining present constantly is hard. Guardians today experience a daily reality such that steady performing multiple tasks is the standard. In making solid family establishments, attempt to be available when your family is talking with you.

Put down gadgets, endeavor to not contemplate the numerous things that you ought to be as of now doing, and effectively stand by listening to everything your loved ones are attempting to say to you. At the point when children are playing, invest energy in their presence, sitting idle yet zeroing in on them.

During feasts, partake in the discussion and company, rather than zeroing in on cleaning counters and washing dishes.

● Set the Model for Youngsters

In the event that you anticipate that your kids should act in a specific way, you should show ways of behaving for them. Families with solid groundworks will pick the ways of behaving and esteems that are essential to them, and model those for more youthful relatives. You can not anticipate that children should be conscious, convey successfully, or be available in others' lives in the event that you, at the end of the day, are not.

- **Opening Impart**

Families with solid groundworks figure out how to transparently and successfully speak with one another.

Conveying really and decidedly helps families in numerous ways like: **Fixing bonds, Figuring out how to trust one another, solving problems, Offering support to one another.**

- **Deliberately Get to know one another**

All lounging around the family room gazing at your gadgets isn't precisely dynamic commitment.

Make reality for yourself as well as your relatives to get to know each other without everyday interruption.

Plan excursions, get-aways, or gadget extra energy to interface with the ones who hold generally dear.

• Building a Strong Ground for Agreeable Living

The strength of a nuclear family is vital in establishing a sustaining and steady climate for our friends and family.

A strong groundwork at home encourages a conviction that all is good and lays the basis for future achievement and satisfaction. I will share a few techniques that have assisted me with building areas of strength for a unit.

By developing trust, making ceremonies, getting together to celebrate, showing appreciation, settling clashes calmly, embracing happiness, advancing energy, focusing on holding exercises, and encouraging a steady climate, we can make a strong nuclear family that will endure for an extremely long period.

Significance of a Solid Nuclear family

The worth of a solid nuclear family couldn't possibly be more significant. It is a place of refuge for each part, giving a feeling of having a place and security.

A strong groundwork at home encourages profound prosperity, advances sound turn of events, and constructs strength in kids.

At the point when relatives feel upheld and adored, they are bound to flourish in all parts of life. Besides, a solid nuclear family is a steady wellspring of inspiration and support, empowering relatives to arrive at their maximum capacity.

By putting time and exertion into building a strong nuclear family, we are laying the foundation for a more promising time to come for our friends and family.

Advantages of a Strong Groundwork at Home

Laying out major areas of strength at home brings various advantages for the two guardians and kids.

It gives a feeling of direction and satisfaction for guardians, realizing they give a sustaining climate to their youngsters to develop.

It fortifies the connection between relatives, encouraging open correspondence and understanding. At the point when difficulties emerge, a strong nuclear family offers a help framework, permitting guardians to explore troublesome times. They are in good company to know them.

A solid groundwork at home imparts a conviction that all is good and fearlessness, empowering kids to investigate the world with a strong base. It makes way for outcome in connections, training, and future undertakings.

CHAPTER 2

Navigating the Challenges and Joys of Raising Children

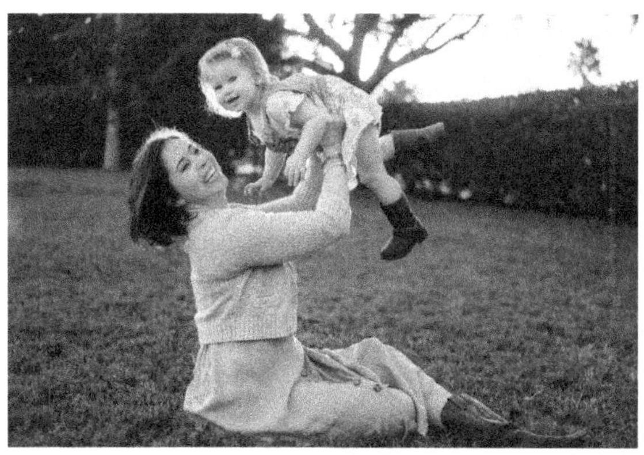

The delight of life as a parent is well established in the bond and association we share with our kids.

From the beginning of snuggling and calming them to the sincere discussions and shared encounters as they become older, these snapshots of association make a feeling of warmth and satisfaction.

As most guardians concur, dealing with a youngster and their many, many requirements can be genuinely and sincerely debilitating.

Regular anxieties, for example, preparing kids for school, telecommuting or getting additional things done, can make nurturing more troublesome.

The genuine delight of bringing up a kid comes from the accomplishment of dynamic nurturing as well as from the individual change you experience through caring affection.

Nurturing is a genuine gift and a major piece of doing life effectively. Embrace it earnestly assuming that you have the open door.

Quite possibly the most difficult thing about nurturing is knowing what's "right." With such a lot of clashing counsel out there, it tends to be difficult to tell what to accept.

In any case, recollect, there's nobody "right" method for nurturing.

You realize your kid best, so pay attention to your gut feelings and make the wisest decision for yourself as well as your loved ones.

5 Methods for beating Your Most prominent Nurturing Difficulties

- Try not to pound yourself.
- Turn your energy toward something you control that will have a positive outcome. Focus on something great.

- Use it to improve.

- Search for the illustration and pass it on.

- Give it to God in a petition.

CHAPTER 3

Partnering for success

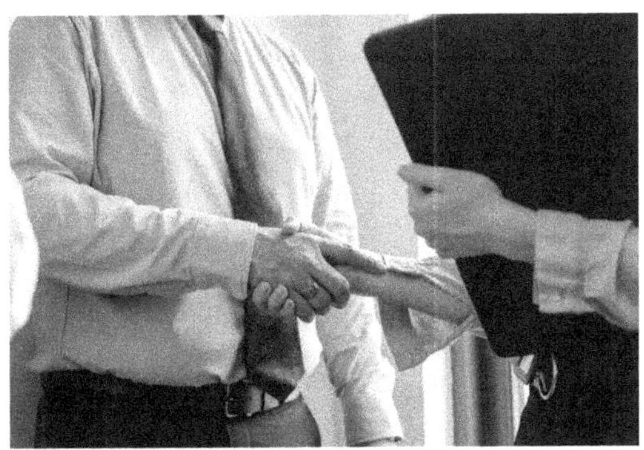

All in all, how would we characterize outcomes in a family? An effective family advances a feeling of good family and individual character, cultivates fulfilling and satisfying connections among all individuals, and adapts to pressure such that outcomes result in additional adaptability and cohesiveness in the family.

Together you can examine the abilities and qualities that every one of you can contribute toward the family's objectives and consider the stressors that might influence the interaction.

These conversations assist us with cooperating to foster techniques and activity ventures for relatives to arrive at their objectives.

Organizations are by definition about individuals cooperating and contacting others to acquire their profound commitment.

Effective associations lay out conventional frameworks to distinguish individuals who can add worth and backing. They decisively construct ties and grow organizations to achieve their needs.

Fortifying the Bond in Your Relationship

In the event that something reinforces a relationship or connection, or on the other hand on the off chance that a relationship or connection fortifies, it makes it closer and bound to keep going for quite a while.

Any sound relationship ought to be established on major areas of strength for a connection. Try to treat your cooperation with a comparable thought, respect, and appreciation as you would a dear companion. Support, pay attention to, and chuckle with one another. Try not to permit yourselves to be impolite or ill bred.

5 Straightforward Ways Of fortifying Your Relationship

- Put away opportunities together.
- Cause normal things to feel more extraordinary.
- Find a side interest or interest that you both can jump aboard with.
- Advise yourself that no family or relationship is great.
- Carve out opportunities to recollect and discuss exceptional minutes in your relationship.

Individuals who need to bond with others , here are a few tips to help:

- Be amicable.
- Center around what you share practically speaking with others.
- Tune in as opposed to talking constantly.
- Keep up with affinity.
- Invest energy with individuals.
- Find and be with individuals who partake in exactly the same things you do.
- Be free when praises are proper.

CHAPTER 4

Effective Communication

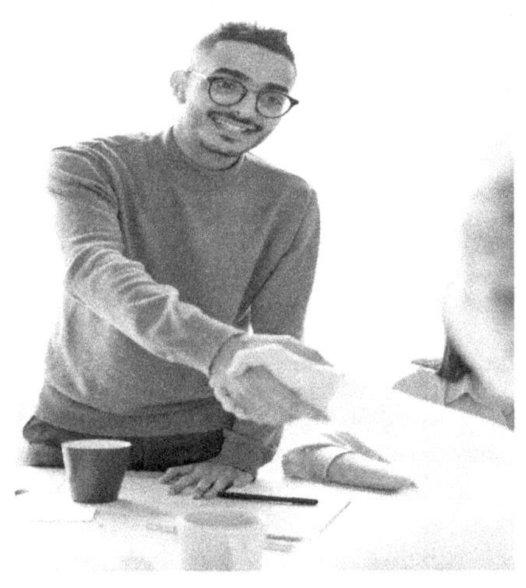

Tranquilly convey your sentiments. Be honest. Listen cautiously to what your kid says.

Utilize your talking times as workable minutes, don't botch valuable chances to show your youngster sound correspondence and how great it tends to be.

How would you convey successfully seeing someone?

Discuss what you need, need and feel - use 'I' articulations, for example, 'I want', 'I need' and 'I feel' acknowledge liability regarding your own sentiments. pay attention to your accomplice.

Set to the side your own contemplations for now and attempt to figure out their expectations, sentiments, needs and needs (This is called sympathy)

One investigation discovered that compelling correspondence expanded relationship fulfillment for couples. 2 Solid correspondence can increase closeness in connections too. The manner in which you and your accomplice speak with one another frequently decides how you settle clashes, so evident.

The key to Understanding and connection

Empathy is a powerful skill that allows us to understand and connect with others on a deeper level. It is essential for building strong relationships, creating a sense of community, and fostering social harmony.

This involves acknowledging and appreciating the feelings, experiences, and opinions of others, even if they differ from our own.

By validating the emotions and perspectives of others, we create a sense of acceptance and understanding. Respect is also crucial in fostering intersubjectivity.

How do I become well connected?

Here are 10 tips to help you build and strengthen connections with people:

- Be your authentic self. You can't go wrong with being yourself.
- Respect people's boundaries.

- Stay focused on the present.

- Move past the surface level.

- Share the conversation.

- Be genuine with your admiration.

- Be a good listener.

- Schedule your time.

CHAPTER 5

Balancing Act

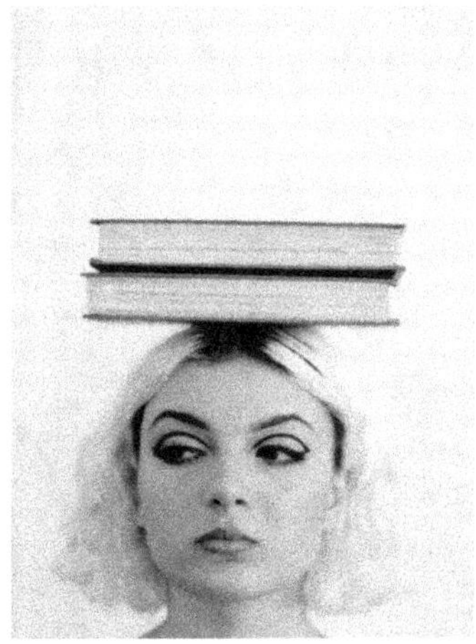

What is going on with the balance act?

An endeavor to deal with or manage at least two things, like commitments all at once to fulfill frequently contending necessities.

This is a significant piece of keeping up with the family, so focus.

For what reason is the difficult exercise significant?

A solid balance between fun and serious activities permits people to keep up with these connections and construct an emotionally supportive network, which can be significant in the midst of hardship.

Besides, a sound balance between serious and fun activities can likewise prompt expanded efficiency and generally speaking position fulfillment.

How would you adjust family work and connections?

- Put forth boundaries.
- Plan and get things done progress of time.
- Arrange flex hours or part time hours if conceivable.
- Go to a movie with your family.
- Find a number two and a number three person.

- Share with other families.
- Limit after-work and after-school involvements.
- Build rituals into your life.
- Take time for yourself and your family.

Overseeing Liabilities and Focusing on Connections.

Focusing on your accomplice just means zeroing in on their requirements and needs seeing someone. Ensure you pay attention to their viewpoints and follow up on them likewise. Cause them to feel appreciated and dealt with.

Focusing on your relationship implies making your accomplice's sentiments, expectations, and dreams as significant as your own.

How might you focus on relationships working in the midst of work requests?

- Distinguish your key connections.
- Plan standard registrations.
- Be available and mindful of your loved ones.

- Follow up and see everything through to completion.
- Set aside a few minutes for your children and accomplice.
- Celebrate and appreciate.
- Learn and get to the next level.

CHAPTER 6

Nurturing Self and Others

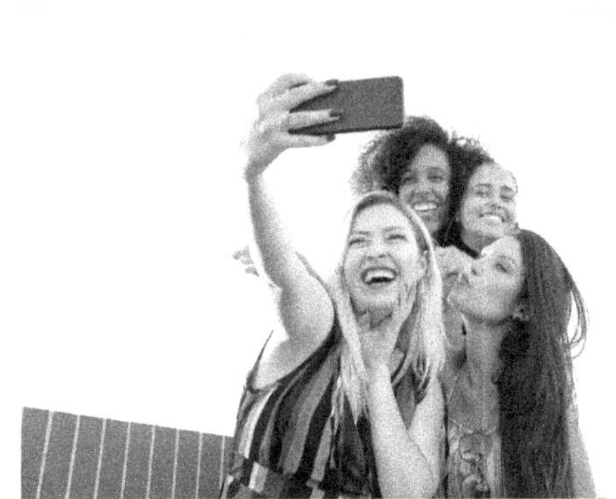

Sustaining yourself as well as other people is tied in with dealing with the physical, mental, profound, and otherworldly necessities.

About taking part in exercises: advance consideration, sympathy, benevolence, and persistence.

Reserving margin for yourself and those you love. Showing adoration and regard is a critical piece of supporting yourself as well as other people.

How would you support an individual?

The following are seven simple propensities that will assist you with sustaining your relationship:

- Correspondence.

- Be Deliberate.

- Show Appreciation.

- Demonstrations of Administration.

- Assume Liability.

- Offer Close to Home Help.

- Excuse and love.

Finding Equilibrium in Personal and Family Growth

Taking time to rest and recharge is vital to help you succeed in what is important to you.

Schedule regular time off for yourself each week to relax, read a book, play sport, spend time in nature or just do nothing. Choose any activity you enjoy.

What are the difficulties of adjusting work and individual life?

Many individuals face difficulties while attempting to adjust work and day to day life requests.

Probably the most widely recognized difficulties incorporate using time effectively, clashing needs, and a requirement for more help from bosses or relatives.

How would you adjust business and family?

7 Different ways to Adjust Everyday Life and Maintaining a Business effectively

- Enroll Delegates at Work and at Home.
- Make a Daily schedule for Yourself (However Consider Adaptability)

- Put forth Objectives consistently.
- Have the option to Adapt to Life's Challenges.
- Be Careful.
- Focus on Family Feasts.

CHAPTER 7

Resilience in Relationships

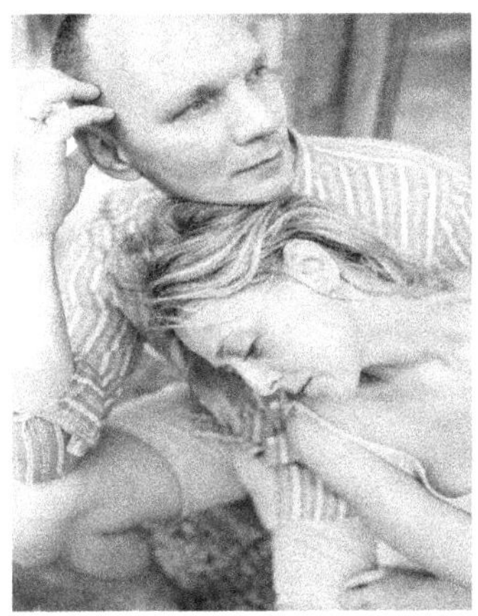

By the very definition, a tough relationship is one that has survived and gained from snags, difficulty, and mishaps and arose more grounded subsequently.

Blossoms and chocolates are perfect (precious stones are far better), however really strong connections are praised with adoration, persistence, and appreciation.

Instances of flexibility abilities

- Good faith: Confidence permits you to zero in on the positive and envision the decency that can result from conditions.
- Persistence.
- Adaptability.
- Mindfulness.

- Put forth objectives.

- Figure out your critical thinking abilities.

- Support your certainty.

- Versatility abilities on your resume.

What are the 8 methods for being strong at difficult stretches?

- Acknowledge what is going on

- Center around things inside your control.

- Acknowledge change by focusing on your past.

- Focus on connections.

- Try not to pull out in difficult stretches.

- Attempt to keep away from gloomy individuals

- Grow your interpersonal organization.

- Get sufficient activity.

Enduring Tempests and Developing All together

What are the tempests in marriage?

Envy and questions over your partner can cause serious tempests in the marriage or courting process.

This happens in light of the fact that a companion female or male might be having a questioning nature or is excessively possessive.

Such ladies and men dishonestly accept their accomplice cheating and has extra-conjugal undertakings.

As a partner, you should construct trust, and figure out how to think before you act

How Couples Can beat any Hardship

- Put your relationship first.

- Fabricate a two-man group.

- Put forth objectives and furthermore set up for difficulties.

- Get master guidance.

- Remember your good fortune.

- Possess understanding and reasoning

- Let love lead

Ways of Exploring Development With Your partner

- Be straightforward with yourselves

- Keep on checking out each other.

- Give Yourself space to become together, furthermore independently.

- Depend on your local area and relationship assets.

- Celebrate (and lament the deficiency of) who you used to be together and as a couple.

- Never listen to gossip.

- Don't be ashamed to face the difficulties together.

CHAPTER 8

Milestones and Celebrations

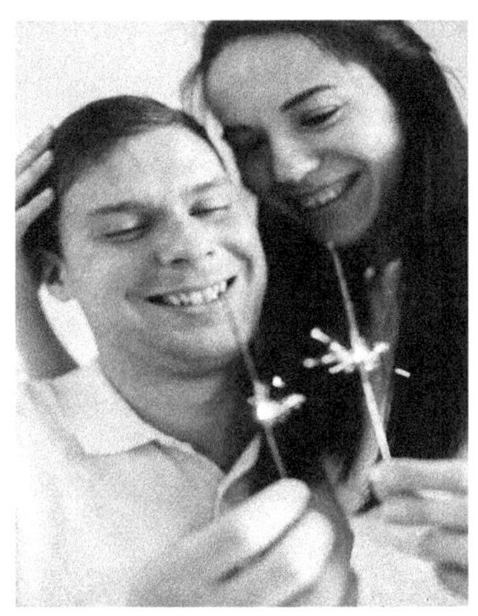

Achievements are huge minutes in our lives that should be praised.

Whether it's a graduation, an advancement, a wedding, or a birthday, these occasions mark another section in our lives and merit remembering with our friends and family.

Ways Of observing Accomplishment

- Simply say it. A direct, eye to eye "great" is a straightforward yet viable method for praising accomplishment.
- Share examples of overcoming adversity.
- Show preemptive kindness.
- Give a gift.
- Get together socially.

- Sort out a day out for yourself as well as your family or companions.
- Offer additional self occasion.

Stamping Snapshots of Adoration and Accomplishment

Perceiving and commending your partner's achievements is central in fashioning a hearty and satisfying relationship. Besides the fact that it shows appreciation for their persistent effort and steadiness, however it likewise grandstands your unflinching help for their desires.

Embracing your accomplice's triumphs contributes decidedly to their identity worth, accordingly enabling them and invigorating your bond.

This affirmation goes beyond anything that can be described, it turns into a demonstration of your common encounters and triumphs, reinforcing your relationship's actual center.

Conclusion

Sustaining Harmony: A Lifelong Pursuit

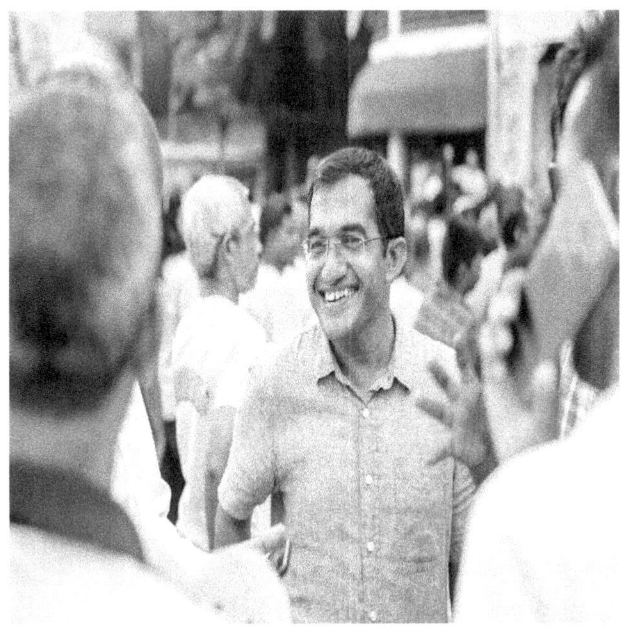

A fulfilling and enriching existence depends on a happy and harmonious family. The idea of family encompasses more than biological ties; it also refers to close ties created by mutual affection, trust, and understanding.

A happy and harmonious family fosters a loving environment where its members can flourish and develop.

As we draw the final curtain on this exploration of parenthood and relationships, it becomes evident that sustaining harmony is not a destination but a lifelong pursuit.

The journey we've undertaken together reveals that the pursuit of harmony involves continual adaptation, unwavering commitment, and an enduring spirit.

In the tapestry of family life, threads of love, communication, and resilience intertwine to create a fabric that withstands the tests of time. It is a fabric woven with shared dreams, cherished moments, and the delicate dance of understanding.

As we navigate the various chapters of our lives, from the early stages of parenthood to the seasoned landscapes of partnership, the pursuit of harmony becomes a guiding principle.

Harmony is not a static state but a dynamic equilibrium that requires constant attention and cultivation.

It thrives on the willingness to learn, grow, and adapt as individuals and as a family unit.

It is in the daily rituals of connection, the shared laughter during moments of joy, and the united front in facing challenges that the symphony of harmonious living finds its resonance. So, as you continue your journey, remember that sustaining harmony is not about achieving perfection but about embracing imperfection with love.

It is about acknowledging that, like any worthwhile pursuit, there will be peaks and valleys, but it is in the commitment to weathering these fluctuations together that true harmony emerges.

May your pursuit of harmony be marked by an abundance of love, a tapestry of shared experiences, and the enduring strength that comes from navigating life's journey hand in hand.

As you step into the ongoing chapters of your story, may the pursuit of harmony be a guiding force, weaving a narrative of fulfillment, growth, and everlasting connection.

www.ingramcontent.com/pod-product-compliance
Lightning Source LLC
Chambersburg PA
CBHW071105260726
48661CB00006B/2467